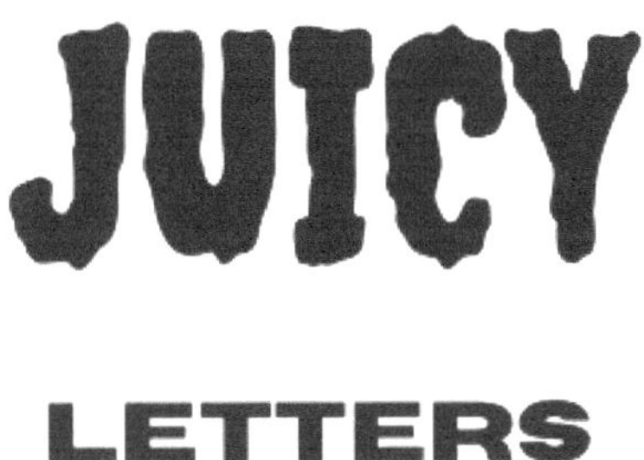

JUICY
LETTERS

AN ALPHABETICAL GUIDE TO FRUITS AND THEIR BENEFITS

SYED MUDASIR MANZOOR

THE BOOK CONTAINS

This book provides important information about 26 different most popular fruits in alphabetical order to make it easy for readers to find information about a specific fruit quickly. Each fruit is accompanied by a page header with an alphabet letter and corresponding fruit name with the scientific name. The description of each fruit includes the edible portion of the fruit, nutritional content, health benefits, best time to eat, largest producer country, and fun facts related to the fruit.

List of Fruits

- **APPLE**
- **BANANA**
- **CHERRY**
- **DATE**
- **ELDERBERRY**
- **FIG**
- **GRAPE**
- **HONEYDEW MELON**
- **INDIAN GOOSEBERRY**
- **JACKFRUIT**
- **KIWI**
- **LEMON**
- **MANGO**
- **NECTARINE**
- **ORANGE**
- **PINEAPPLE**
- **QUINCE**
- **RASPBERRY**
- **STRAWBERRY**
- **TANGERINE**
- **UGLI FRUIT**
- **VELVET APPLE**
- **WATERMELON**
- **XIGUA**
- **YANGMEI**
- **ZUCCHINI**

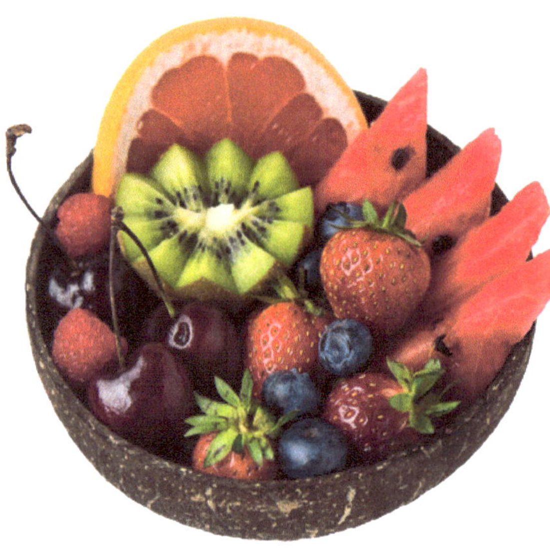

INTRODUCTION

Welcome to "Juicy Letters: An alphabetical guide to fruits and their benefits"! This book is a comprehensive guide to the numerous health benefits and nutritional content of fruits.

The purpose of this book is to provide readers with a complete alphabetical guide to fruits and their benefits,from A to Z. Eating a variety of fruits is an essential part of a healthy diet, and this guide will help you discover new fruits to add to your diet while also highlighting the benefits of the ones you already love.

Fruits are a vital component of a healthy diet, providing essential vitamins, minerals, and nutrients that the body needs to function properly. Eating a variety of fruits hasbeen linked to numerous health benefits, including a reduced risk of heart disease, stroke, and some types of cancer.

This book is organized in alphabetical order to make it   easy for readers to find information about a specific fruit quickly. Each fruit is accompanied by a page header with analphabet letter and corresponding fruit name with the scientific name. The description of each fruit includes theedible portion of the fruit, nutritional content, health benefits, best time to eat, largest producer country and fun facts related to the fruit.

Whether you're a fruit lover looking for new ideas or someone who wants to learn more about the health benefits of fruits, "Juicy Letters" is the perfect guide to help you make informed decisions about the fruits you choose to include in your diet.

"Juicy Letters: An alphabetical guide to fruits and their benefits" can be beneficial for a wide range of age groups. However, it is particularly useful for children and young adults who are developing healthy eating habits, as well as anyone interested in learning more about the health benefits of various fruits.

For children, the book provides an engaging and informative way to learn about different fruits and their nutritional value, which can help encourage healthy eating habits from an early age. The fun facts and descriptions can also make learning about healthy foods more enjoyable and memorable for kids.

For young adults and adults, the book can serve as a handy reference guide for choosing nutritious and delicious fruits to incorporate into their diet. The information on health benefits, nutritional content, and best time to eat can also help readers make informed decisions about their food choices.

Overall, "Juicy Letters" can be a valuable resource for anyone looking to learn more about fruits and their benefits, regardless of age.

 APPLE

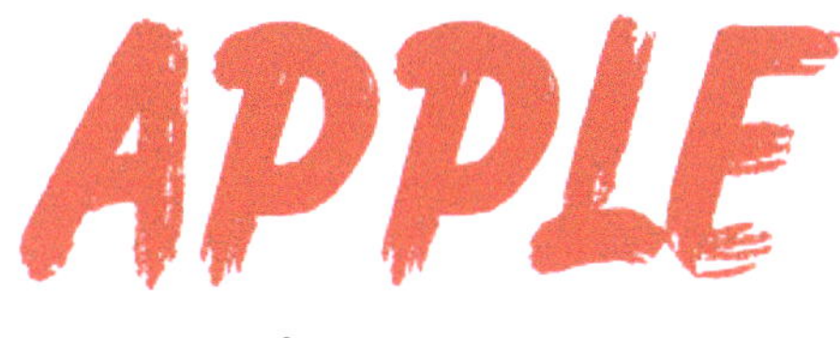

(Malus domestica)

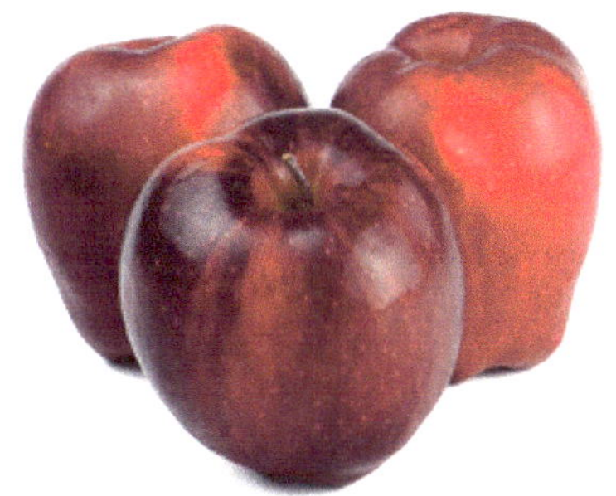

KNOW THIS!

Edible portion: The edible portion of an apple is the flesh, which is surrounded by the skin and seeds.

Nutritional content: Apples are a great source of Fiber, Vitamins-(C,K,A) and Antioxidants like Flavonoids & Phenolic compounds. They also contain small amounts of minerals such as Potassium, Calcium, Magnesium & Iron.

Health benefits: Regular consumption of apple has been linked to a lower risk of chronic diseases such as Heart disease, Type 2 diabetes, and certain cancers. The fiber in apples can also aid digestion and promote satiety, helping to control appetite.

Best time to eat: Apples are accessible year-round, yet the pinnacle season is in the fall (September-November) when they are fresh.

Largest producer country: China is the largest producer of apples, followed by the United States.

Fun facts: There are over 7,500 apple varieties grown worldwide. Apples float in water because 25% of their volume is comprised of air.

BANANA

(*Musa acuminata*)

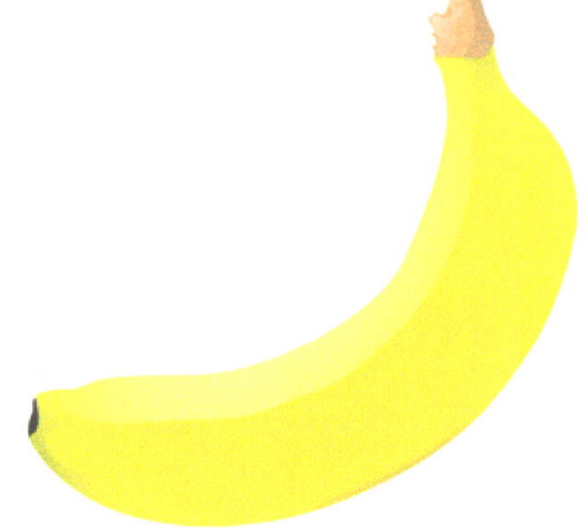

KNOW THIS!

Edible portion: The edible portion of a banana is the fruit, which is encased in a soft, yellow or green skin.

Nutritional content: Bananas are a good source of Fiber, Potassium, Vitamin C, Vitamin B6, and Antioxidants. They are also low in Fat and Calories.

Health benefits: Bananas can help lower blood pressure and reduce the risk of heart disease. They may also help improve digestion, boost energy levels, and regulate blood sugar.

Best time to eat: Bananas are available year-round. One should ideally consume them in the morning or the evening and must avoid eating them at night.

Largest producer country: India is the largest producer of bananas, followed by China and the Philippines.

Fun facts: Bananas are technically Berries. A cluster of bananas is called a "Hand", while a single banana is called a "Finger". They contain a natural chemical called 'Serotonin', which makes people happy.

CHERRY

(Prunus avium)

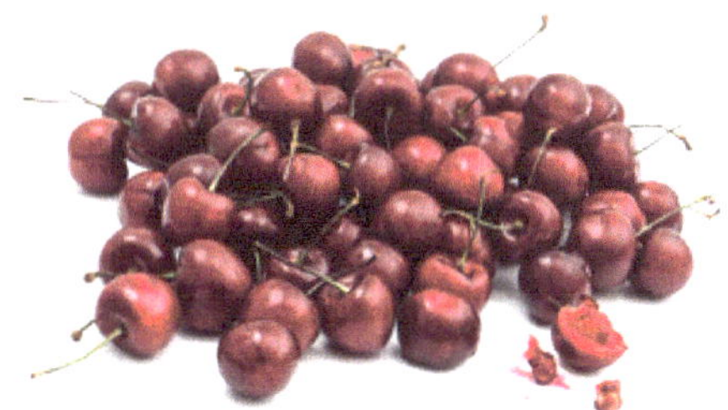

KNOW THIS!

Edible portion: The edible portion of a cherry is the fleshy fruit, which surrounds a hard pit or stone.

Nutritional content: Cherries are a good source of Fiber, vitamin-C, Potassium and antioxidants. They are low in calories, fat & Protein. They have a large concentration of beneficial 'Phytonutrients' that have positive effects.

Health benefits: Cherries help to reduce inflammation, prevents Gout by restoring normal Uric acid levels, improves sleep and lowers the risk of heart disease & colon cancers. They also help relieve pain and soreness associated with exercise and muscle damage.

Best time to eat: Cherries are typically in season from May to August. They should be consumed before sleep as it contains Melatonin which helps to get a good night's sleep.

Largest producer country: Turkey is the largest producer of cherries, followed by the United States and Iran.

Fun facts: The red pigment in cherries, called anthocyanin, is also responsible for the color of other fruits like blueberries, grapes, and eggplants. Cherries can cause cancer cells to commit suicide.

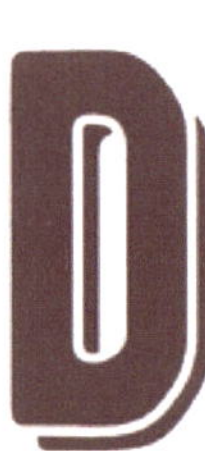
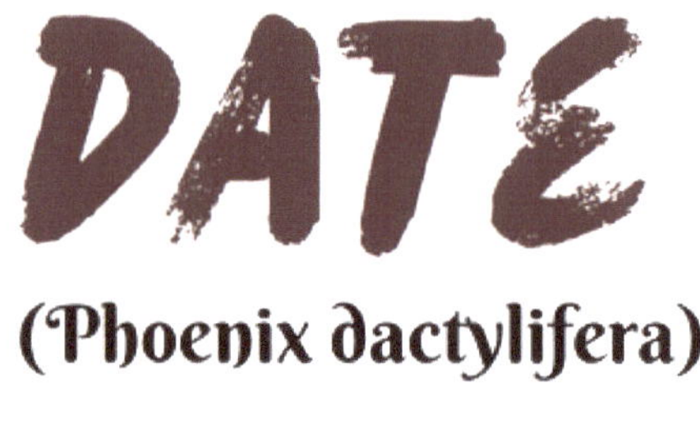

DATE
(Phoenix dactylifera)

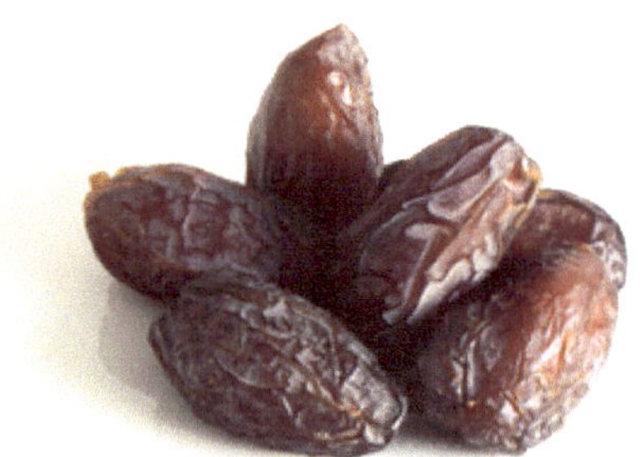

<u>Edible portion</u> : The edible part of the date is the sweet, fleshy fruit that surrounds the seed.

<u>Nutritional content</u>: Dates are a good source of energy, fiber, and essential minerals like potassium, magnesium, and iron. They also contain six B vitamins and vitamin K. They also have a high concentration of 'Polyphenols' a potent antioxidant.

<u>Health benefits</u>: Dates have an impressive "free-radical" scavenging ability & antitumoral activity. They have several health benefits such as improve digestion, reduce blood pressure, lower risk of heart disease, promote strong bones, reduce Menopausal symptoms etc.

<u>Best time to eat</u>: Dates are commonly eaten as a snack or as a dessert after a meal.
<u>Largest producer country</u>:   The largest producer of dates is Egypt.

<u>Fun facts</u> : Dates have been cultivated for over 6,000 years and are mentioned in religious texts such as the Bible and the Quran. They are also known as the "bread of the desert."

ELDERBURRY

(Sambucus nigra)

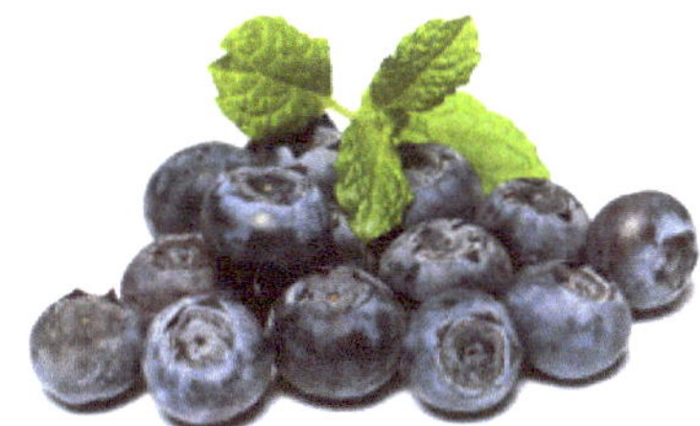

KNOW THIS!

Edible portion: The edible part of the elderberry is the dark purple/black berry.

Nutritional content: Elderberries are a good source of antioxidants, vitamins A and C, fiber and calcium.

Health benefits: Elderberries help in boosting the immune system, help in fighting Colds & Flu, reduce inflammation, assist in weight loss, help in relieving constipation and improving heart health.

Best time to eat: Elderberries are typically used to make jams, jellies, syrups, and wine. They can be consumed at any time of day.

Largest producer country: The largest producer of elderberries is Bulgaria.

Fun facts: Elderberries have been used for medicinal purposes for centuries, and the flowers and berries are often used in traditional medicine to prevent potential cancers.

F   *FIG*

(Ficus carica)

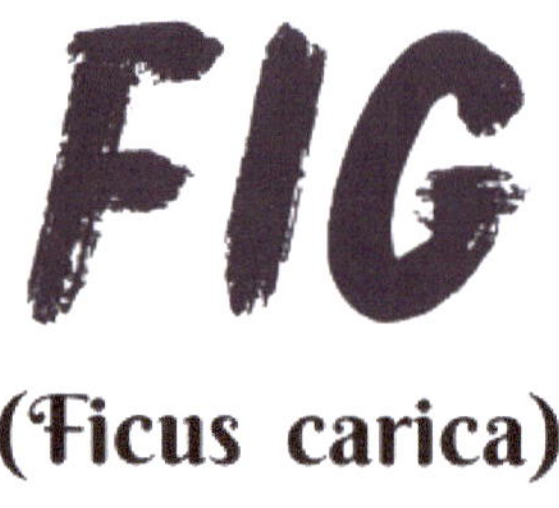

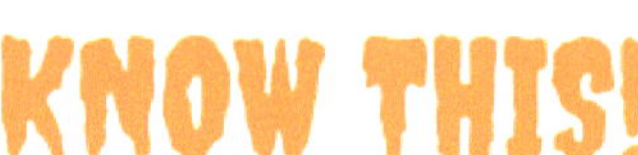

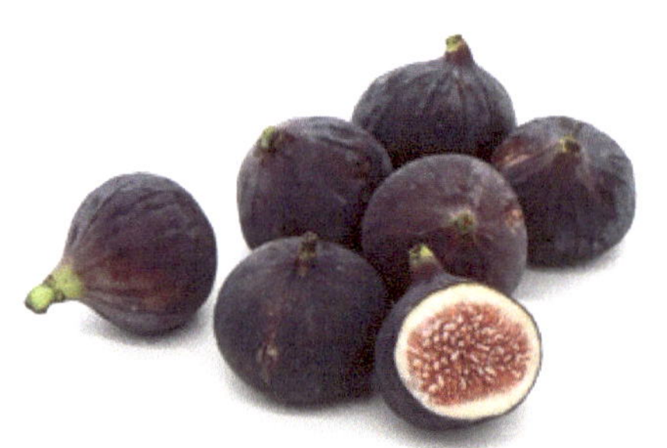

Edible portion: The edible part of the fig is the fleshy, sweet fruit that surrounds the seeds.

Nutritional content: Figs are a good source of fiber, Copper, potassium, and calcium. They also contain vitamins B6 and K.

Health benefits: Figs have been associated with several health benefits such as improved digestion, decrease constipation, lower blood pressure, manage blood fat and sugar and reduce risk of heart disease.

Best time to eat: Figs are typically eaten fresh or dried as a snack or used in recipes. The optimal time to consume them is in the morning on empty stomach.

Largest producer country: The largest producer of figs is Turkey.

Fun facts: Figs are one of the oldest cultivated crops, dating back to ancient civilizations such as the Greeks and Romans. In some cultures, figs are seen as a symbol of fertility and prosperity.

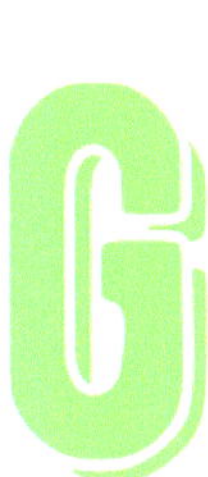 GRAPE

(*Vitis vinifera*)

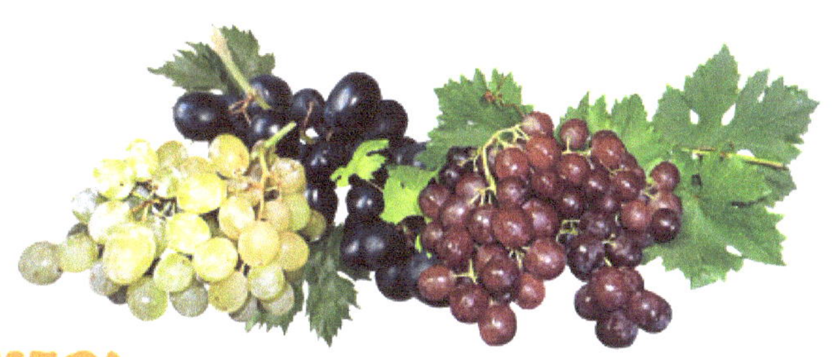

KNOW THIS!

Edible portion: The edible part of the grape is the juicy fruit that surrounds the seeds.

Nutritional content: Grapes are a good source of antioxidants, vitamins C and K, and fiber.

Health benefits: Grapes have been associated with several health benefits such as improved heart health, lower blood sugar levels, and reduced inflammation.

Best time to eat: Grapes are typically eaten fresh as a snack, used in recipes, or used to make wine.

Largest producer country: The largest producer of grapes is China.

Fun facts: Grapes come in a variety of colors such as red, green, and black. They are also one of the oldest cultivated crops, dating back to ancient civilizations such as the Egyptians and Phoenicians.

HONEYDEW

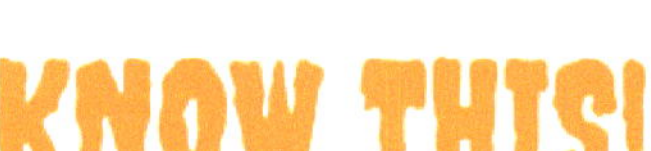

(Cucumis melo)

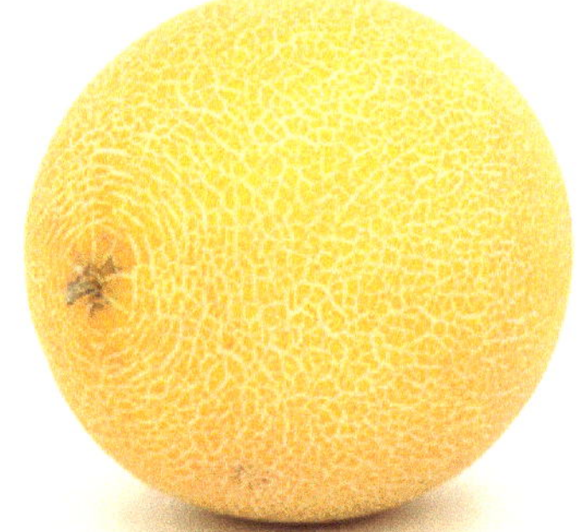

KNOW THIS!

Edible portion: The edible portion of the honeydew melon is the flesh, which is juicy and sweet.

Nutritional content: Honeydew is low in calories and a good source of vitamin C, potassium, folate, magnesium and dietary fiber.

Health benefits: Eating honeydew may help in preventing Neural Tube Birth Defects, protects against Vision loss, promotes Skin and heart health and acts as anti-dehydrating agent.

Best time to eat: Honeydew is best enjoyed in the summer when fully ripe. They act as 'perfect pre-bedtime' snack.

Largest producer country: China is the largest producer of honeydew melons, followed by Turkey and Iran.

Fun facts: Honeydew is a member of the Cucurbitaceae family, which also includes cucumbers and watermelons. It is believed to have originated in Africa and was first cultivated in ancient Egypt.

INDIAN GOOSEBERRY

(Emblica officinalis)

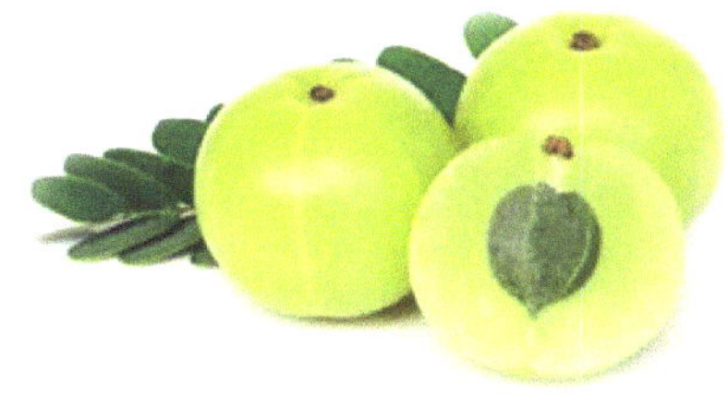

KNOW THIS!

Edible portion: The edible portion of the Indian gooseberry, also known as amla, is the fruit pulp and seeds.

Nutritional content: Indian gooseberries are a rich source of vitamin C, antioxidants, and minerals like calcium, phosphorus, and iron.

Health benefits: Eating Indian gooseberries may help improve digestion, boost immunity, and promote healthy hair and skin.

Best time to eat: Indian gooseberries are available in the winter season and are best eaten when they are ripe and fully grown.

Largest producer country: India is the largest producer of Indian gooseberries, followed by Sri Lanka and Nepal.

Fun facts: Indian gooseberries are highly valued in Ayurvedic medicine and are used to treat a variety of ailments, including diabetes, respiratory disorders, and liver problems.

J JACKFRUIT

(Artocarpus heterophyllus)

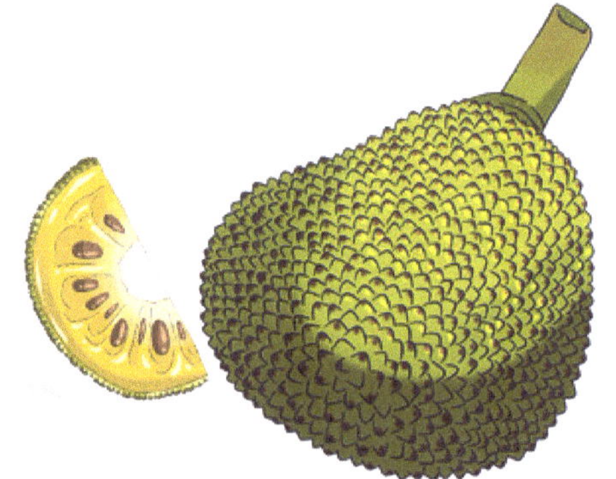

KNOW THIS!

Edible portion: The edible portion of jackfruit is the flesh or arils, which can be eaten ripe or unripe.

Nutritional content: Jackfruit is a good source of vitamin C, dietary fiber, and potassium, and contains small amounts of vitamin A and minerals like magnesium, manganese & copper.

Health benefits: Eating jackfruit helps to improve digestion, boost immunity, regulate blood sugar, prevents calcium loss from bones, prevents Anemia and improves vision.

Best time to eat: Jackfruit is best enjoyed when it is fully ripe and has a sweet flavor. Unripe jackfruit is often used as a meat substitute in vegetarian dishes.

Largest producer country: India is the largest producer of jackfruit, followed by Bangladesh and Thailand.

Fun facts: Jackfruit is the largest tree-borne fruit in the world and can weigh up to 80 pounds. It is also a popular ingredient in vegan and vegetarian dishes because of its meat-like texture.

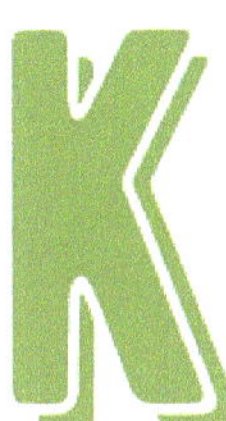

KIWI
(Actinidia deliciosa)

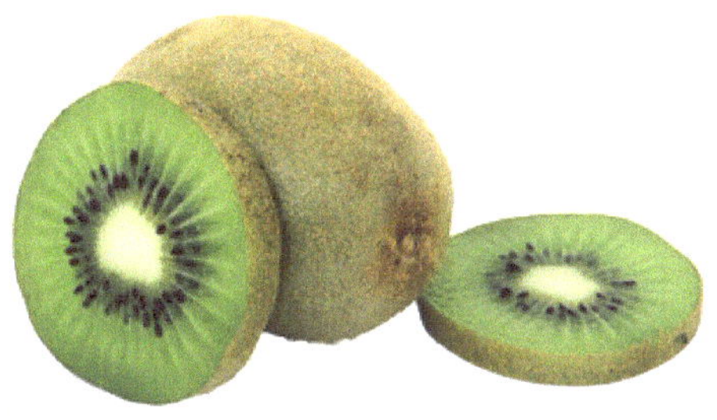

KNOW THIS!

Edible portion: The edible part of Kiwi fruit is the flesh inside, which is soft and juicy, with small edible seeds.

Nutritional content: Kiwi is a rich source of Vitamin C, dietary fiber, and potassium. It also contains antioxidants like lutein and zeaxanthin.

Health benefits: Kiwi is good for digestion, immune system, and cardiovascular health. It can also aid in weight management and improve skin health.

Best time to eat: Kiwi can be eaten any time of the day but it is better to consume it on an empty stomach or before meals to aid in digestion.

Largest producer country: China is the largest producer of Kiwi, followed by Italy and New Zealand.

Fun facts: Kiwi was originally known as the Chinese Gooseberry and was first grown in China. It was later brought to New Zealand and renamed as Kiwi, after the national bird of New Zealand.

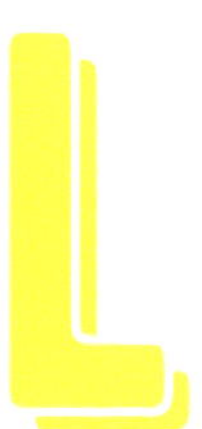
LEMON
(Citrus limon)

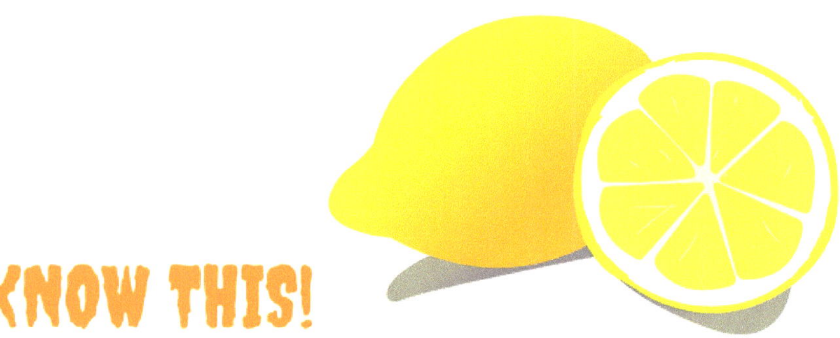

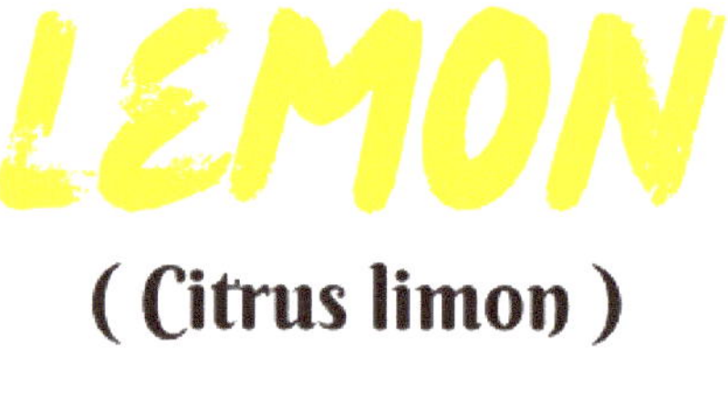

KNOW THIS!

<u>Edible portion:</u>   Edible part of Lemon fruit is the pulp and the juice.

<u>Nutritional content:</u> Lemon is a rich source of Vitamin C, dietary fiber, and citric acid. It also contains antioxidants like limonene and flavonoids.

<u>Health benefits:</u> Lemon is good for digestion, immune system, and skin health. It can also aid in weight loss and reduce the risk of heart disease.

<u>Best time to eat:</u> Lemon can be consumed any time of the day. It is often used as a flavoring agent in drinks and food.

<u>Largest producer country:</u> India is the largest producer of Lemon, followed by Mexico and China.

<u>Fun facts:</u> Lemon trees can produce up to 600 pounds of lemons per year. The juice of Lemon can be used as a natural cleaner and disinfectant.

MANGO
(Mangifera indica)

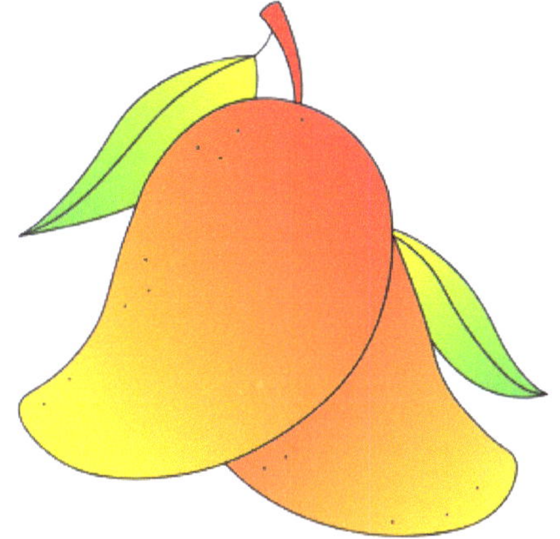

Edible portion: The edible part of Mango fruit is the pulp inside, which is sweet and juicy.

Nutritional content: Mango is a rich source of Vitamin C, Vitamin A, dietary fiber, and potassium. It also contains antioxidants like beta-carotene and lutein.

Health benefits: Mango is good for digestion, immune system, and eye health. It can also aid in weight loss and reduce the risk of certain cancers.

Best time to eat: Mango can be consumed any time of the day. It is often eaten as a dessert or used as a flavoring agent in dishes.

Largest producer country: India is the largest producer of Mango, followed by China and Thailand.

Fun facts: Mango trees can grow up to 100 feet tall and produce fruit for up to 300 years. The Mango is the national fruit of India, Pakistan, and the Philippines.

N NECTARINE

(Prunus persica)

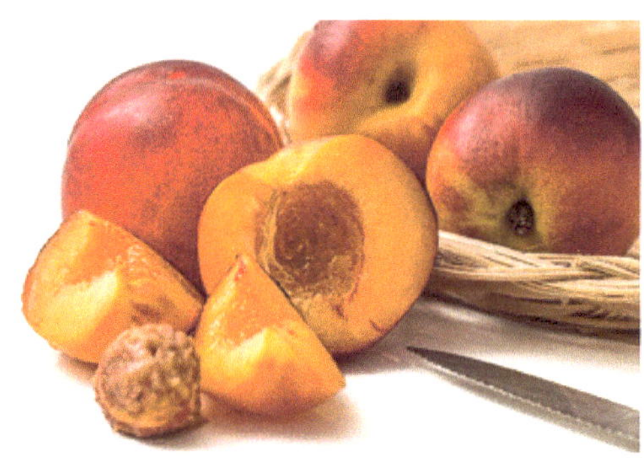

KNOW THIS!

Edible portion: The edible portion of a nectarine is its juicy, sweet flesh.

Nutritional content: Nectarines are a good source of vitamins A and C, potassium, and dietary fiber.

Health benefits: Nectarines can help boost your immune system, improve digestion, and promote healthy skin.

Best time to eat: Nectarines are best eaten when they are fully ripe, which is typically in the summer months.

Largest producer country: China is the largest producer of nectarines, followed by the United States and Italy.

Fun facts: Nectarines are actually a variety of peach that have a smooth, fuzz-free skin. They are believed to have originated in China over 2,000 years ago.

O | ORANGE

(Citrus sinensis)

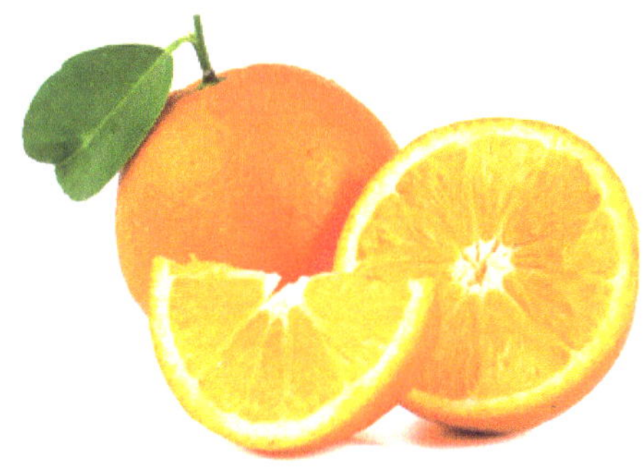

KNOW THIS!

Edible portion: The edible portion of an orange is its juicy, pulpy segments.

Nutritional content: Oranges are a good source of vitamin C, folate, and potassium. They also contain bioactive compounds like Flavonoids(Hesperidin, Naringenin) and Carotenoids (lycopene, beta-cryptoxanthin).

Health benefits: Oranges can help improve immune function, lower cholesterol, reduces the risk of some chronic diseases, enhances iron absorption and supports heart health.

Best time to eat: Oranges are best to be consumed on an empty stomach, in the morning for breakfast, after resting or as a snack between main meals.

Largest producer country: Brazil is the largest producer of oranges, followed by the United States and Mexico.

Fun facts: Oranges were originally a hybrid of pomelo and mandarin fruits. They are a popular ingredient in many cuisines around the world.

PINEAPPLE

(Ananas comosus)

KNOW THIS!

Edible portion: The edible portion of a pineapple is its juicy, fibrous flesh.

Nutritional content: In addition to Vitamin C and Manganese, Pineapples contains Vitamin B6,Copper, Thiamine, folate, Potassium, magnesium, Niacin, Riboflavin and Iron.

Health benefits: Pineapples can help reduce inflammation, aid digestion, ease symptoms of Arthritis and boost immunity.

Best time to eat: Pineapples are typically in season during the summer months, but they can be found in stores year-round.

Largest producer country: Costa Rica is the largest producer of pineapples, followed by the Philippines and Brazil.

Fun facts: Pineapples are actually a type of bromeliad plant. They contain the Bromelain enzyme which can breakdown proteins, so can be used to tenderize meat.

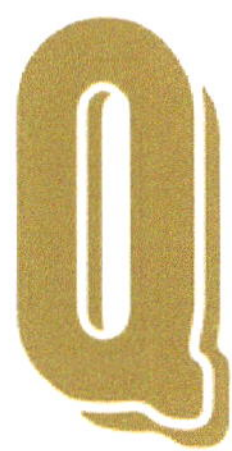

QUINCE
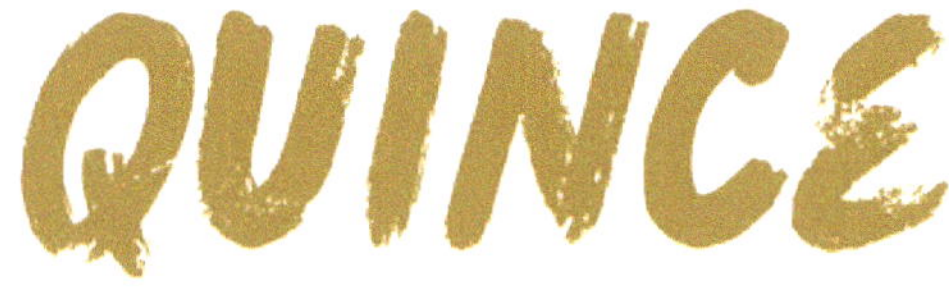
(Cydonia oblonga)

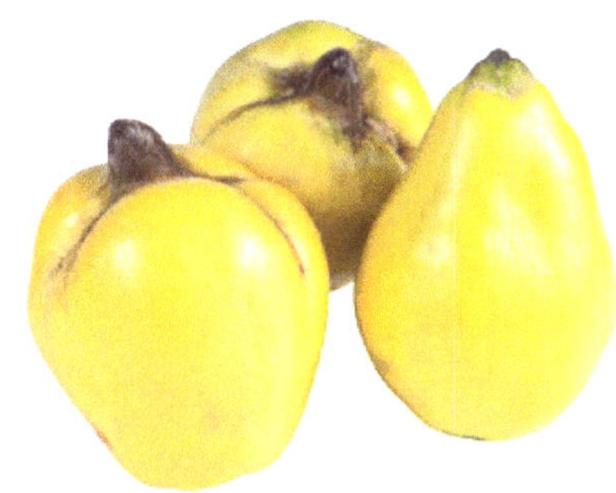

KNOW THIS!

Edible portion: The edible portion of a quince is its firm, tart flesh, which is often used to make jams and jellies.

Nutritional content: Quinces are a good source of vitamin C, B1, B6, Copper, Iron, Potassium, Magnesium, dietary fiber, and antioxidants.

Health benefits: Quinces can help improve digestion, aids in IBS symptoms, decreases Acid reflux, helps with Morning sickness, support immune function, and promote healthy skin.

Best time to eat: Quinces are typically in season during the fall months.

Largest producer country: Turkey is the largest producer of quinces, followed by Iran and Azerbaijan.

Fun facts: Quinces have been grown for thousands of years and were a favorite fruit of the ancient Greeks and Romans. They are often used as a symbol of love and fertility in mythology and folklore.

RASPBERRY

(Rubus idaeus)

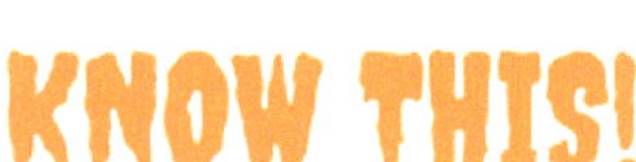

KNOW THIS!

Edible portion: The edible portion of raspberry is the fruit, which is composed of many small juicy drupelets that form around a central core.

Nutritional content: Raspberry is an excellent source of dietary fiber, vitamin C, and manganese. It also contains significant amounts of vitamin K, vitamin E, and folate.

Health benefits: Raspberry has antioxidant and anti-inflammatory properties, which can help protect against chronic diseases such as cancer and heart disease. It also supports healthy digestion and may help lower blood sugar levels.

Best time to eat: Raspberries are typically in season during the summer months, from June to September. They are best eaten when fully ripe and can be enjoyed fresh or used in a variety of desserts, jams, and sauces.

Largest producer country: The largest producer of raspberries is Russia, followed by the United States, Poland, and Serbia.

Fun facts: The name "raspberry" comes from the Old French word "raspe," which means "a thicket."

STRAWBERRY
(Fragaria ananassa)

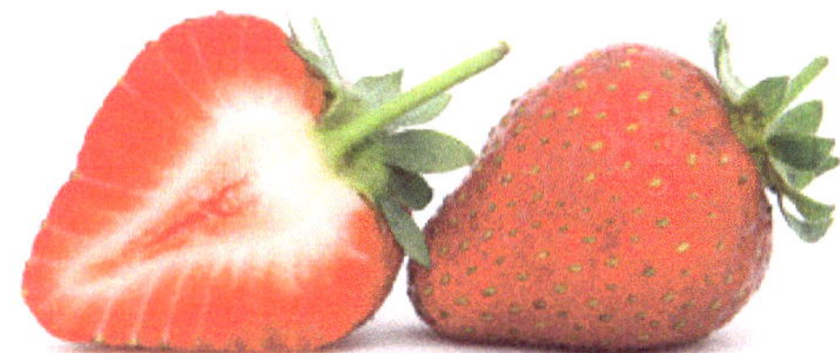

KNOW THIS!

Edible portion: The edible portion of strawberry is the fleshy, red fruit that is covered in tiny seeds.

Nutritional content: Strawberry is a good source of vitamin C, manganese, and folate. It also contains significant amounts of dietary fiber, potassium, and antioxidants.

Health benefits: Strawberry has been shown to have anti-inflammatory and anti-cancer properties. It may also help lower blood sugar levels and improve heart health.

Best time to eat: Strawberries are in season during the summer months, from June to August. They are best eaten when fully ripe and can be enjoyed fresh or used in a variety of desserts and sauces.

Largest producer country: The largest producer of strawberries is the United States, followed by Spain, Mexico, and Turkey.

Fun facts: Strawberry is the only fruit that has its seeds on the outside. It was first cultivated in France in the 18th century by crossing two wild strawberry species.

TANGERINE
(Citrus reticulata)

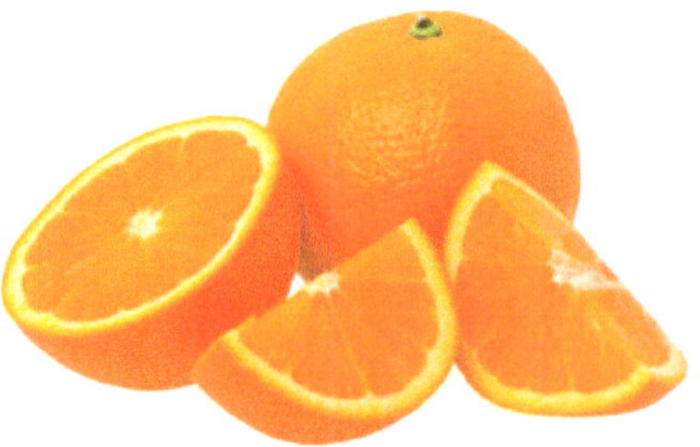

Edible portion: The edible portion of tangerine is the juicy, pulpy fruit that is covered in a thin, easy-to-peel skin.

Nutritional content: Tangerine is a good source of vitamin C, vitamin A, and folate. It also contains significant amounts of dietary fiber, potassium, and antioxidants.

Health benefits: Tangerine has been shown to have anti-inflammatory and anti-cancer properties. It may also help lower cholesterol levels and improve heart health.

Best time to eat: Tangerines are in season during the winter months, from November to April. They are best eaten when fully ripe and can be enjoyed fresh or used in a variety of desserts and salads.

Largest producer country: The largest producer of tangerines is China, followed by Spain, Turkey, and Egypt.

Fun facts: Tangerines are a type of mandarin orange and are often referred to as "mandarins" in some countries. They are named after the city of Tangier in Morocco, where they were first imported to Europe.

U UNGLI FRUIT
(Diospyros peregrina)

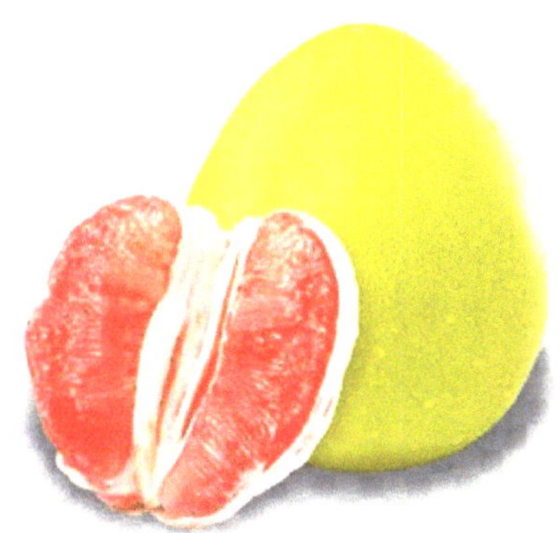

Edible portion: The edible portion of the Ungli Fruit is the pulp surrounding the seed, which has a sweet and tangy flavor.

Nutritional content: The fruit is a good source of vitamin C, iron, calcium, and phosphorus.

Health benefits: The fruit is known to boost immunity, aid digestion, and improve skin health.

Best time to eat: Ungli fruits are best eaten when fully ripe, which is indicated by the fruit turning a bright yellow or red color.

Largest producer country: The Ungli Fruit is native to South and Central America, and is commonly grown in countries like Brazil, Colombia, and Mexico.

Fun facts: In some parts of South America, the fruit is used to make a popular beverage called "Spondias", and the wood of the Ungli tree is often used to make furniture.

VELVET APPLE

(Diospyros blancoi)

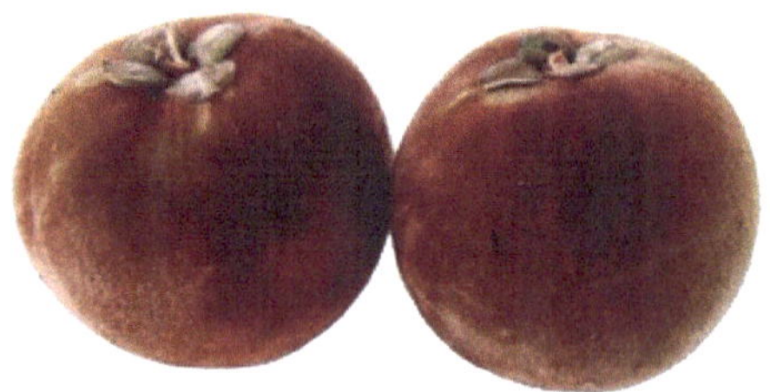

KNOW THIS!

Edible portion: The Velvet Apple is a round fruit with a soft, velvety skin and a juicy, sweet flesh that is eaten raw.

Nutritional content: The fruit is a good source of vitamin C, potassium, and fiber.

Health benefits: The Velvet Apple is known to aid digestion, boost immunity, and lower cholesterol levels.

Best time to eat: The fruit is usually harvested when it is fully ripe and the skin has turned a deep reddish-brown color.

Largest producer country: The Velvet Apple is native to the Philippines and is commonly grown in Southeast Asian countries like Thailand, Indonesia, and Malaysia.

Fun facts: The fruit is often used in traditional medicine to treat various ailments, and the leaves of the Velvet Apple tree are used to make a natural dye.

WATERMELON

(Citrullus lanatus)

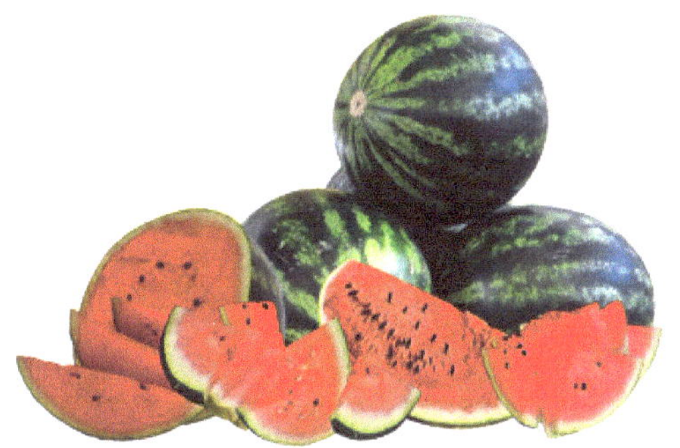

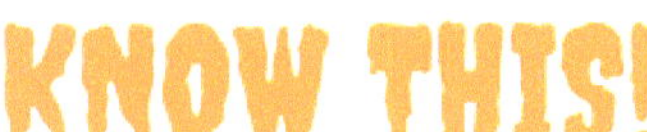

Edible portion: The edible portion of watermelon is the juicy flesh inside the fruit. The seeds are also edible and can be roasted or ground into a paste.

Nutritional content: Watermelon is a great source of vitamin C, vitamin A, and potassium. It is also low in calories and contains high amounts of water, making it a great choice for hydration.

Health benefits: Watermelon has numerous health benefits, including improving heart health, reducing inflammation, and helping to prevent cancer. It is also great for skin health and can improve digestion.

Best time to eat: Watermelon is best eaten during the summer months when it is in season and at its sweetest.

Largest producer country: China is the largest producer of watermelon, followed by Turkey and Iran.

Fun facts: Watermelon is actually a member of the cucumber family and is considered a fruit and a vegetable. The heaviest watermelon on record weighed over 350 pounds!

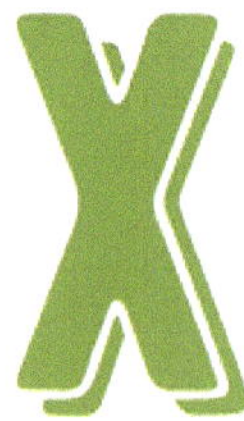

XIGUA

(Citron melon)

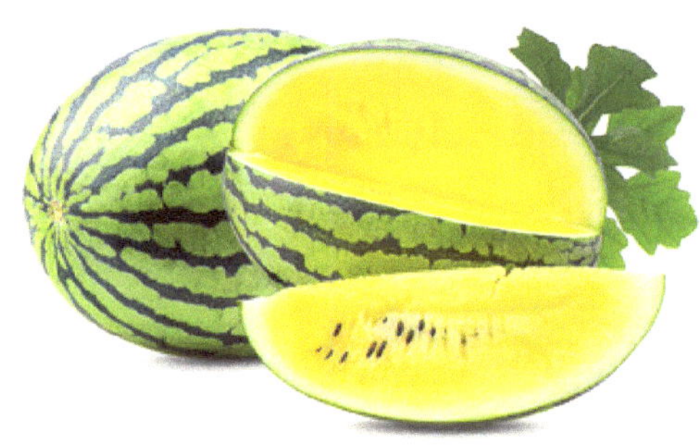

<u>Edible portion:</u> The edible portion of xigua is the sweet and juicy flesh inside the fruit. The seeds are also edible and can be roasted or ground into a paste.

<u>Nutritional content:</u> Xigua is a good source of vitamin C, potassium, and fiber. It is also low in calories and contains high amounts of water.

<u>Health benefits:</u> Xigua has numerous health benefits, including improving digestion, reducing inflammation, and promoting healthy skin. It is also great for hydrating the body and can help to lower blood pressure.

<u>Best time to eat:</u> Xigua is best eaten during the summer months when it is in season and at its sweetest.

<u>Largest producer country:</u> China is the largest producer of xigua.

<u>Fun facts:</u> Xigua is also known as the Chinese watermelon and is a popular fruit in China, where it is often eaten during the Dragon Boat Festival.

YANGMEI
(*Myrica rubra*)

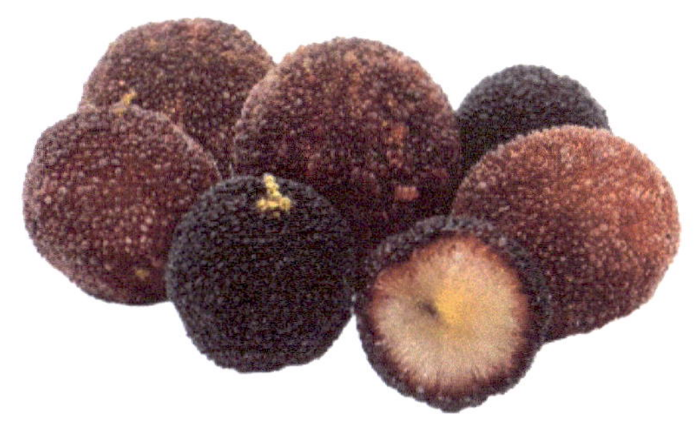

KNOW THIS!

Edible portion: The edible portion of yangmei is the sweet and tangy flesh inside the fruit. The seeds are not edible and should be removed before eating.

Nutritional content: Yangmei is a good source of vitamin C, vitamin E, and antioxidants. It is also low in calories and contains high amounts of fiber.

Health benefits: Yangmei has numerous health benefits, including improving heart health, reducing inflammation, and promoting healthy skin. It is also great for boosting the immune system and can help to lower blood pressure.

Best time to eat: Yangmei is best eaten during the summer months when it is in season and at its sweetest.

Largest producer country: China is the largest producer of yangmei, followed by Taiwan.

Fun facts: Yangmei is also known as the Chinese bayberry and is a popular fruit in China, where it is often used in desserts and drinks.

ZUCCHINI

(Cucurbita pepo)

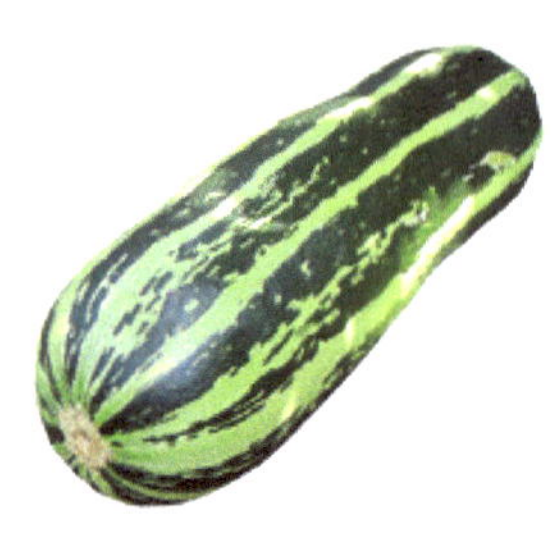

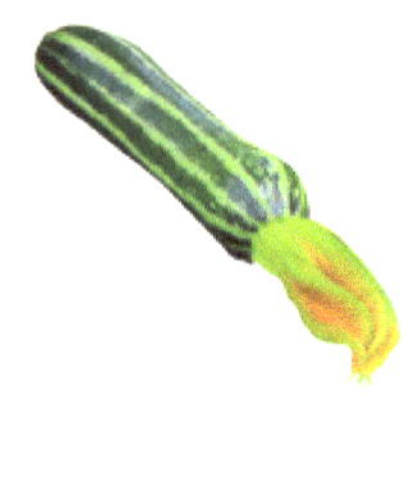

KNOW THIS!

Edible portion: The entire zucchini is edible, including its seeds, skin, and flesh.

Nutritional content: Zucchini is low in calories and high in dietary fiber. It also contains several essential nutrients such as vitamins A, C, and K, potassium, and folate.

Health benefits: Zucchini is known for its anti-inflammatory properties and may help in reducing the risk of chronic diseases such as heart disease and cancer. It may also aid in digestion, improve eye health, and boost the immune system.

Best time to eat: Zucchini is a summer squash and is best consumed during the summer months when it is in season and readily available.

Largest producer country: China is the largest producer of zucchini in the world, followed by Turkey and Italy.

Fun facts: Zucchini is technically a fruit, but it is commonly referred to as a vegetable due to its culinary uses. The word "zucchini" comes from the Italian word "zucchina," which means "small squash." Zucchini flowers are also edible and are often used in Italian cuisine

CONCLUSION

In conclusion, "Juicy Letters: An alphabetical guide to
fruits and their benefits" is a comprehensive guide to the
numerous health benefits and nutritional content of fruits.
Eating fruits is an essential part of a healthy diet, and this guide has highlighted
the importance of incorporating a variety of fruits into your diet. Fruits provide
essential vitamins, minerals, and nutrients that the body needs to function
properly, and eating a variety of fruits has
been linked to numerous health benefits.

As you've learned from this book, there are many different types of fruits
available, and each has its unique benefits. I encourage you to try new and
different fruits, experiment with recipes, and find new ways to incorporate fruits
into
your diet.
Incorporating a variety of fruits into your diet can provide numerous health
benefits, including a reduced risk of heart disease, stroke, and some types of
cancer. It can also help you maintain a healthy weight and provide energy
throughout the day.

In conclusion, I hope this book has been a helpful guide to discovering new fruits
and learning about the benefits of the ones you already love. Remember, a healthy
diet is all about balance, so keep enjoying those juicy fruits!